Pacing for Pain

Control Your Pain, Reclaim Your Life

BY JONATHAN BLOOD SMYTH

Dustjacket Books

Published by Dustjacket Books

12 The Moorings, Victoria Road, Exmouth, EX8 1DY, UK

First published by DustJacket Books 2014

Printed by CreateSpace

ISBN 978-0-9538065-2-2

About the Author

JONATHAN BLOOD SMYTH B.Sc. (Hons) Zoology, Grad. Dip. Phys., MCSP, is an HCPC Registered Physiotherapist in the United Kingdom. He qualified as a physiotherapist from Leeds School of Physiotherapy in Leeds, UK, in 1982.

After working at Addenbrooke's Hospital in Cambridge, UK, he moved to the Princess Elizabeth Orthopaedic Hospital in Exeter UK. There he specialised in the assessment and management of orthopaedic and musculoskeletal conditions.

From 1997 he specialised in the assessment and management of pain conditions. He was part of the Pain Management Therapy team at the Royal Devon and Exeter Hospital, Exeter, UK.

From 2010-2014 he was physiotherapy consultant to a Health Care Management Company.

Publications include:

• Co-author of an abstract on the costs of manipulation

• Co-author of a paper on the back pain service in Exeter

• Author of the booklet “Total Knee Replacement. A guide to getting the best from your new knee” First published 1995.

• The Physiotherapy Site at www.thephysiotherapysite.co.uk

His work interests include rehabilitation, joint replacement and pain management. Other interests include natural history, computing, wine and Formula One.

Visit JonathanBloodSmyth.com to contact Jonnie

Disclaimer

BECAUSE WE ARE unaware of any pre-existing health conditions you should consult with your doctor or a qualified medical practitioner before using or practising any of the methods described in this book.

The information provided in this book is designed to provide helpful information on the subjects discussed. This book is not meant to be used, nor should it be used, to diagnose or treat any medical condition. For diagnosis or treatment of any medical or musculoskeletal problem, consult your own physician and/or physiotherapist as appropriate.

The publisher and author are not responsible for any specific health needs that may require medical supervision and are not liable for any damages or negative consequences from any treatment, action, application or preparation, to any person reading or following the information in this book.

References are provided for informational purposes only and do not constitute endorsement of any websites or other sources. Readers should be aware that the websites listed in this book may change.

Preface

THIS BOOK CAME from meeting a marathon man with a problem. He told me "I can't run for more than 15 minutes before my back becomes so painful I have to stop".

That's what the fit, somewhat unhappy 54 year old man was saying was his problem. He had been a runner since he was a young man and had competed in several marathons. He still ran twenty miles in one session at least once a week.

Well he used to.

His back pain had come on steadily about three months before and this had started to cut into his running and become a nuisance. Every time he went out running he felt fine for the first 15 minutes then BANG, his back pain came on significantly, forcing him to stop.

He'd repeated this unrewarding pattern regularly for the last month but his back pain was just as bad and his running had not improved. He was getting fed up with the restrictions and had begun to ask himself "Should I give up running?".

As a physiotherapist of 22 years experience, working with a Pain Management Team for 10 years, I look for technical reasons for a person's pain and do technical things to them.

Except I didn't.

I explained the reasons for his pain and how his behaviour was maintaining the problem. I suggested he changed his running technique to take account of "pacing" to control his pain.

It worked. Three months later he came back to report on this progress. He had taken a month to get back to twenty mile runs but he had done it. Then he fell down a bank in a garden at night at a party! This made his back worse, but he had moved up to twenty miles again over the next four weeks.

The pacing system had worked for him twice in three months!

To be honest it wasn't just this man that started my interest in pacing, but it was his very clear story that made me think about writing something for everyone with pain problems. The principles apply to many people and in many different situations. I felt that this knowledge could be useful.

I hope you find it so.

Jonathan Blood Smyth

Exmouth August 2014

1

Pacing for Pain

Introduction

IN THIS BOOK I discuss the role of activities in pain conditions. I aim to give you a clear path to reduce your pain and increase your ability to do normal things.

Pain is an important and common problem in adults but is not well catered for in medicine. I was a physiotherapist attached to a Pain Management Team for over ten years. We saw thousands of patients with a wide variety of pain conditions.

One of the things which struck me most forcefully was the role of activities in pain problems. Activities are important because that's much of what life consists of, doing things we have to do or want to do.

Pain limits what we can do but activities can be a main cause of pain and its persistence.

Pain is always a problem in itself. However many people accept their pain and are more distressed that they can't do their normal activities.

I do not address the whole problem of chronic pain. I have noted some references under "Resources" towards the back of the book which have a wider scope. I haven't focussed just on chronic pain either. I will also cover activities which can cause acute (recent) pain such as overdoing sport or an unfamiliar chore.

I will explore information about pain, activities, behaviour and change to help you understand the reasoning behind the Pacing System.

Understanding "the reasons why" makes us more likely to keep on with something once we have started. If you've had your pain for some time then waiting a little longer to read through this book makes sense.

How to use this book

This book is meant to help you. How you use it is up to you but I thought I'd give you a few pointers.

If you have the time and patience, read the book all the way through. It's meant to be read that way and holds together in the order I've set down.

If you're in a real hurry to get started then you can go straight to the chapter "How to Pace" and get going right away. But you might be more successful if you first read the chapters "The 5

Principles of Pacing" and especially "The Six Traps". The traps are really sneaky at catching you out so it's worth knowing about them beforehand.

In the appendices you can find shortened versions of what I've covered in the book. They allow you to see the sequence of actions needed to succeed. I have also given an example there to show you the kind of working out that's necessary for the best results.

2

What is the Pacing System?

Managing Our Activity

THE PACING SYSTEM is an effective way of managing your activity so it does not cause you pain or increase pain which already exists.

People with chronic pain problems complain more about the restriction of their activities, not being able to join in with life, rather than about the pain itself.

We all fall into typical patterns of activity to try to achieve our goals and those habits can serve us well. But our habits can also serve us badly.

I will describe the typical patterns of activity and the traps we fall into again and again. I will outline a method of managing our activities which stops winding the pain up and allows us to do more with time rather than less.

I will show you just how simple it is to apply the Pacing System to your life. This can really make a difference to your pain and to your ability to get things done.

I will point out the traps just waiting to sabotage your progress and to put you back at square one again and again. And how to get round each one to ensure your success.

Who Can Benefit?

Everyone can benefit from this information!

Yes, I mean it. Every single one of us could benefit from this technique, at least at some stage of our lives.

I wrote this because I spent my daily working life trying to help people with chronic pain problems. But I have come to realise that the principles you will be learning apply to us all. It doesn't matter how young or how fit you are, the Pacing System applies.

• Do you dig the garden?

• Do you have a job which requires physical work?

• Do you play sport or take part in a physical activity?

• Have you ever had an operation or injury and took a while to recover?

• Do you have a pain problem of some kind which

limits your physical abilities?

• Does your pain limit your ability to do your job?

If you can answer “Yes” to any of these questions then these ideas apply to you.

Most athletes take these principles for granted when training or getting back into shape after a lay-off. The better they are at pacing, the fewer problems with injury they are likely to have and the more success at their chosen event. Even so, I bet some of them overdo things and suffer setbacks.

Most of us non-athletes can cope well with sudden increases in activity. We can do spring cleaning or unexpected chores with only moderate discomfort. However, if we go for it we can start off a problem which may remain with us for years.

If you already suffer pain it’s a different case altogether. The results of overdoing can be severely out of proportion to the activity you performed. Massive increases in pain can result, causing a sharp drop in your activity and an increase in low mood and anxiety.

How can I benefit best from this information?

I think the most important thing here is to have an open mind. Some of my suggestions will seem odd to you and you may find it a challenge to put my ideas into practice. But they are tried and tested with hundreds of people.

I ask you to consider the idea of pacing as an experiment, which you can run with for a while and not lose anything. If it works well, great. If you find it doesn't help, you haven't lost anything.

You have bought this book because things are not going as well as you wish and your life is not as you want. You'd like to change things for the better. You've gone as far as to buy my product, so don't waste it, have a go at some of the following advice.

I suggest you read through the whole book first so you get an view of the overall idea and plan before you try and make changes. A good understanding of chronic pain and the reasons for doing what I suggest is important before you set off.

What Pacing Can Do for You

The best way to find out how the Pacing System can benefit you is to get in there and try it out for yourself. But if you want a preview without getting off the couch, here are a couple of real examples from my practice. They illustrate the kind of problems people have and how the Pacing System can help.

A Very Determined Lady

"I've just got to keep on going and get things done", said the 44 year old lady sitting in front of me with a six year history of back and leg pain. She used to be slim, fit and able to do all the things she wanted to. Since her back problem she had gained weight, lost her fitness and found her activities restricted by pain. She was frustrated by this.

On assessment her behaviour was part of the problem which maintained her pain state. I taught her the principles of the Pacing System and sent her away for four weeks.

"I'm 90% better!", was the amazed response one month later when I asked her how it was going. She had really got hold of the theory and practice of pacing and completely changed the way she did things. It worked. And how!

One month later she rated herself close to 100% better, so much happier and feeling in control of her life.

John and the Grass

It was John's job to mow the grass, and that was always fine with him. It was part of his manly role in life. Until, that is, he developed chronic (long-term) back pain and everything became more complicated.

He felt it was still his role to do the grass. Knowing it would be difficult, he went at it and stuck it out until the job was done. Unfortunately, his back pain was then so bad he could do little for the next few days.

John and I went through the Pacing System and I tried to make it relevant to him so he could achieve what he wanted without too many problems.

Pacing did not make everything wonderful for John. But it helped him to do one of his important duties without the severe consequences.

The examples I have given are real people who came to consult me about their back pain problems. Amongst other things, I recommended pacing as part of the plan so they could manage their pain problems. They all felt significant benefit.

What Pacing Will Not Do

1. Cure your pain. Unfortunately this rarely occurs if you have a significant pain problem. If there was an answer to your pain you'd likely have had it by now.

2. Make everything wonderful. Pacing is only a way of managing your pain, although it can be very powerful. You will need to use other methods too.

3. Motivate you if you lack this. You have to commit yourself to changing your behaviour for this technique to be useful. This is harder than it looks.

4. Allow you to get back to normal levels of activity. If you have a chronic pain problem it is likely your activity levels will remain limited for a person of your age. Pacing can help a lot but it can't make you brand new.

3

Pain

Introduction

WE'RE ALL FAMILIAR with pain. If we're lucky we get pain only when we injure ourselves, learn our lessons and go back to our normal, pain-free state. Pain is doing its job and we steer clear.

Pain is confusing and complicated. Many of the things we think we understand about pain are just plain wrong. This can lead us to make poor decisions when we inevitably come up against a pain problem of some kind.

Research in neuroscience has shown how pain systems work and how our brains process this kind of incoming sensation. Pain medicine has expanded into an important medical specialty even though there is still much we do not know.

This chapter covers the reasons for pain, its biological function, acute pain, chronic pain and the important differences between the last two. That should set us up for understanding what happens when we get pain.

The Function of Pain

We have pain for a reason. Evolution would not have equipped us with pain unless we really, really needed it. In fact pain is vital for our survival and the few people who are born without being able to feel pain do not have good or long lives.

Pain is a sophisticated alarm system which protects us from further injury. This maximises our chances of returning to our normal selves as soon as possible.

When we cut ourselves or hit ourselves hard against an object we are immediately aware of the intensity and place of the pain. The brain interprets the incoming pain signals and tells us that we have injured our thigh by whacking it against the side of a table. This way we can check the area for visible damage and take action according to the severity of injury.

Pain sets off two kinds of body alarms:

• **The urgent alarm**, telling us to move away at once to prevent further damage. The instant flinching we perform when our fingers touch a too-hot object is a good example. We can't control this, our hand just withdraws from the heat at great speed. This alarm is important but less so than the next one.

• **The slow alarm**, letting us know something serious has occurred and that we need to do something about it. This alarm continues for some time as the aching pain which often comes after the sharp pain of the injury. This is the brain's way of limiting our activity until healing has progressed far enough to start using the damaged part again.

Pain's reason for existence is to help ensure our survival. It restricts our normal movement and limits the length of time we spend in stressful positions.

Pain is forcing us to protect the damaged area until it has the opportunity to heal. Pain limits further damage by stopping us doing the same activity again before the injured area has settled.

There's no negotiation with the pain of injury, it commands and we obey.

Acute Pain

Acute pain is recent. And short term. If you've just cut yourself, just sprained your ankle or just got a tooth abscess, you are suffering acute pain. Acute pain can be severe but does not have to be. You could get a mild headache and because it's recent, it's an acute pain.

Acute pain is our brain's way of making us aware of the signals from recently injured body tissues. A key part of this is the inflammatory response to tissue injury. Damaged cells in the injured area release inflammatory chemicals. This increases the sensitivity of nearby pain nerves which fire off much more easily and more often.

This huge increase in pain nerve firing from the injured part heads up towards the central nervous system. When it gets there it causes trouble. The nerves in the spinal cord which receive the incoming pain signals become hypersensitive. This means they fire off much more easily, sending pain quickly up towards our conscious mind.

I call this increase in pain levels the pain amplifier. It is important both in our normal reactions to injury and in the more long-term pain problems we will look at later.

Let's look at what happens when you sprain your ankle.

The Useful Pain of Ankle Sprain

Ouch! Over it goes, you've sprained your ankle. You know the feeling, it starts with a jolt of severe, sharp pain which brings you up quickly and makes you hop on the other leg. As the severe pain goes off, it's replaced by a duller, throbbing, unpleasant pain which persists.

When you damage your ankle ligament, the injured cells release powerful "injury chemicals" into the local area. These chemicals are kinins and prostaglandins. They make the local nerve endings much more sensitive and more likely to fire off.

Nerve endings in the damaged areas are now firing off much more easily than normal. The injury chemicals wind them up so they fire more and more. These chemicals also wake up nerves which don't usually respond much and make them sensitive too.

This is what we call acute pain.

So what do you do? If you're anything like me, you stop what you're doing and look after your injury. Perhaps you will limp home or get someone to give you a lift. You lie on the sofa with your leg up, take painkillers or anti-inflammatories and put ice on your ankle.

You might wear a compression dressing to control the swelling and reduce the amount of time you spend on your feet for a while.

As we've seen, in medicine acute pain is not defined by the type of pain you are suffering, it refers to how long you've had it.

Acute pain is recent and it's useful.

It stops you doing stupid things like continuing your previous activity and damaging your ankle badly. It's your protective shield, your guarantee that you will get better if you obey the rules.

Acute pain means you have damaged yourself, and if you continue, then further tissue damage may result. In these cases, pain equals damage.

Pain Equals Damage

"Pain equals damage" is how we usually think when we hurt. We assume we have injured part of our body and take appropriate action. This point is important later.

That all looks pretty straightforward, doesn't it? Despite the complexity of all kinds of pain, it is. Let's look at all the things you know about this incident.

What We Know About Acute Pain

IT'S TIME TO review a few things about acute pain so we can compare them to chronic pain. The differences are very important and greatly affect how we go about helping people in pain.

• **You know how you did it**. It's a cut, a sprain or a blow and the level of pain and problems is closely related to the severity of the injury.

• **You know when you did it**. We can usually place when we caused ourselves an injury, or when an accident occurred.

• **You know what has happened (more or less)**. We may not understand the detail of exactly what has happened but we do know a good amount. We know what a cut, a sprain or a blow mean in general terms.

• **You know how to treat it**. We are all experts in treating acute pain from experience. We rest and take painkillers. We put ice on it, bandage the ankle, avoid aggravating activities and elevate the injured part.

• **You know roughly how long the problem is likely to last**. We don't know we're going to be better at 11 o'clock next Wednesday. But we do know, more or less, that in a certain time we are likely to be back to normal.

• **You know you will get better**. We may not think about it, but we firmly expect the injury to settle and to go back to our normal level of function.

That's a lot of things to be sure about, and it is comforting to know this.

This story of acute pain is well known and we treat it naturally without much thought. The point comes when we start to think about chronic pain, where all the rules change and nothing is at it seems.

Chronic Pain

Chronic pain is very common. Half of all adults suffer from either persistent (long term) or recurrent (repeated) pain of some kind. These are both chronic pain. This can vary from the severely disabling pain of cancer or arthritis to the mild pain of an old injury to a joint or ligament. Doctors can diagnose some pains and the treatments are clear.

But many pains have no diagnosis and no treatment.

This includes most back and neck pain, migraines, headaches, many abdominal pains and a number of pain problems without a diagnostic label.

Chronic pain is a severe burden on an individual, his or her partner and children, their work, the medical services and the state.

It can turn an independent member of society into an inward-looking, isolated person. It can make them dependent on the state for money and on their family and friends for care.

If you have any of these problems you will already know what I mean. Are you truly in control of your life? Do you want greater control over your life and greater independence?

This book will tell you, step-by-step, how to get out of the rut you have found yourself in. You can move towards regaining independence and a more fulfilling life.

The Nature of Chronic Pain

Now you've got the acute pain idea straight, let's move on to the hard stuff. To understand chronic pain we need to do a bit of neurophysiology.

Don't panic, even though it's a little tricky to understand it's well worth it. A new way of understanding can make a huge difference. Suddenly you will look at pain in an entirely different manner, gaining new insights and new ways of coping and managing.

Think back to my previous explanation about acute pain. So when acute pain comes in from the excited nerves in the damaged area it flows unchanged straight up to the brain, right?

No, that's not what happens at all.

The nerve carrying the incoming pain signals ends in the spinal cord and passes its signals to a second nerve. This will take them on up towards the brain. If the signals are strong enough they will "jump" the gap to the second nerve and progress on up.

However, that is not all the incoming signals do to the second nerve. Flooded with wave after wave of incoming pain signals, the second nerve starts to change. And these changes can have profound consequences for our future.

The second nerve activates previously dormant genes which start to make new chemicals in the nerve. These chemicals are called neurotransmitters. They are special agents which change the electrical and chemical behaviour of any nerve they are in contact with.

The bottom line is that the second nerves become much more sensitive to incoming pain signals. They amplify them before they get sent on upwards to the brain. They wind themselves up and go a bit mad.

Imagine you've just injured your back and your injury is suddenly sending 50 units of pain up the nerves towards your spinal cord.

(Please note I am making these figures up! 50 units of pain doesn't really make sense, but it's useful to illustrate what's going on.)

Anyway, these 50 units of pain are firing off regularly from your irritated nerves in the area of damage. They make their way up the nerve pathways. 50 – 50 – 50 – 50 – 50, the second nerve receives these messages and begins to change. One 50 would be no big deal, but a whole wagon-train of them is another thing entirely.

The second nerve starts to respond more and more strongly to the incoming messages. It increases its output as the incoming pain streams in.

50 – 50 – 50 ok so far…….

But then it starts to output 100, 200, 500, 1000, 5000. Ouch! Now's the time you stop doing whatever it was and take notice of your pain. Some of the pain you are feeling is coming from irritated nerves in the damaged area and some is from the second nerve amplifier.

The Amplifier

That’s what I call it. Inside the spinal cord is an amplifier which can greatly increase the incoming signals as it passes them on up towards the brain.

What’s the point of that? I think it’s a survival thing, a way of stopping ourselves from keeping on going and damaging ourselves. Our ankle nerves may not produce enough pain alone to make us take notice and do something we don't want to, like stop playing football and rest.

If the pain was only mild or moderate in intensity you might continue to do whatever caused the injury in the first place. This would cause increasing tissue damage and make you less likely to “survive”.

The amplification in the spinal cord happens every time we have an injury or pain and is part of the normal reaction of the nervous system.

So if it always occurs then why don’t we all have serious pain problems then?

In normal cases, when we have a pain problem there are lots of “good” incoming nerve signals to counteract the pain impulses. These impulses come down from the brain and from normal body structures reacting to movement and pressure as we move about.

As time goes on, the injured area begins to settle and the pain impulses coming in decrease. With "good" incoming impulses from other areas this helps the second nerves calm down to their normal settings. The amplifier resets itself gradually back to its normal level.

But not always. Sometimes the amplifier gets stuck.

Imagine you get home from being out for the day and decide you want to listen to some music. You put your favourite CD on and it's loud! So you turn it down but it won't work. It's still loud.

You look at the amplifier and see that it's stuck at 6. You can turn it up and shake the house but you can't turn it down beyond 6, so you have to listen to it loud. Chronic pain is like that.

Pain messages coming in to your spinal cord may be mild or moderate like the signals from the CD to your amplifier. The output, what you feel, is much, much higher. It's like your nervous system amplifier is stuck on 6.

And if the second nerves become super-sensitive to incoming signals they may amplify everything. This could include many different types of messages coming in from the painful area. In this way even normal feelings can feel like pain.

Have you noticed that? If someone prods you in the back or you bump against something, or even in some cases if the area is touched lightly, you get a pain? This is what happens when your nervous system goes into overdrive and winds up all the messages it gets.

Is There a Point to Chronic Pain?

If pain is supposed to be a warning sign, what use is chronic pain?

There's no point to chronic pain!

Your body always tries to correct itself towards normal function and normal chemical makeup. If your water content drops, your blood becomes more concentrated. Your brain then tells you to drink water to bring things back to normal.

Now let's take an injury. If you injure yourself the body responds to the damage by forcing you to take the actions necessary to get back to normal.

The pain minimises any activity that will pose a risk to recovery and remains long enough until the injury is safely on its way to healing. After the healing process has moved along enough the pain withdraws and lets the normal function of the area return.

Our bodies tell us what to do all the time, and if we take notice of it things usually go well. Whatever is wrong settles slowly back to normal, to within the normal range for us.

So if this is the way things are, pain should tell us what to do and when we do it, we should get better. Yep, that's about it.

Except it doesn't work at all for chronic pain.

Your pain tells you there is something wrong and you respond:

• You rest

• You keep going

• You try and push through the pain barrier

• You take anti-inflammatory tablets to calm the injury

• You have treatment with a chiropractor, osteopath or physical therapist

• You attend numerous doctors and have numerous diagnoses and suggested investigations and treatments

You do all these things, led by the messages from

your pain. And what's the result of all this? Nothing. No change at all. Absolutely no effect.

What We Know About Chronic Pain

Let's look at all the things you know about acute pain, but apply them to chronic pain instead:

• **You don't really know how the chronic pain developed**. You may have had an accident or some kind of event which started your pain initially but how did it change into what it is now?

• **The levels of pain you get seem to be out of proportion** to what you have done

• **You don't know when you did it**, when you caused your problem. When did it start getting this bad?

• **You don't know what has happened inside your body**. You can imagine what happens when you damage yourself but not when you have a continual pain which doesn't "heal".

• **You don't know how to treat it**. You've tried tons of different drugs, therapies and goodness knows what else, to no effect.

• **You don't know how long the problem is likely to last**. Normal pains settle down pretty quickly but yours has gone on for ages and that doesn't seem right.

• **You don't know if you will get better**. Surely it will settle down at some time? But you don't know and that's worrying.

If we look at this list we can see that nothing we know about acute pain holds true for chronic pain. Everything is different, all the rules have changed and there's no instruction booklet for the new game.

If you are using what you know about acute pain to try and deal with chronic pain, that just won't work. We need a new plan to cope with this very different world where the acute pain rules don't apply.

Before we get to the plan we need to cover activities and their effects on body tissues.

4

Activities and Pain

Doing Things

A PSYCHOLOGIST I used to work with says human life consists of three things: thoughts, feelings and activities (behaviour). I've tried to think of something that doesn't fit into those categories but haven't been able to so far. So maybe she's right!

I will cover attitudes, beliefs, mood and thoughts another time. Here I concentrate on the effect on the third main aspect of life, activities..... doing things.

We all have to do things, want to do things and are expected to do things. We may have a job, do housework, look after children, have hobbies, travel, have duties. These all need a certain degree of physical ability to perform.

Often we pay no attention to the fact that our bodies do all these amazing things without complaining. That is, until something happens which interferes with our body's abilities.

Pain always interferes with physical activity and not just the activities mentioned above. If the pain is bad enough, things we take for granted may be greatly restricted. This can include sitting, standing, walking and sleeping.

Yes, we all have to accept a reduction in our physical abilities as we get older, but pain can bring it on much sooner than we expected.

Suddenly we are much less able than we expected to be for a person of our age. We can see people of our age and much older easily managing the tasks we cannot.

Pain is invisible so other people cannot see the problems you have. This makes them less likely to make allowances than for someone with a broken bone.

You may feel obliged, as you look fit and healthy, to do things you know are going to be a problem for you. You may feel self-conscious and embarrassed when you cannot help. Someone may look at you and see a younger, stronger person than themselves.

This can lead to going out less and less to avoid the need to explain or expose yourself to others' point of view.

You don't go out to the pub or for a meal, or visit people in case you get asked to do something or have to spend too long in one position. You may feel embarrassed about getting up or telling anyone about your problems. Who wants to always hear about someone's problems? You might well think this and find it hard to walk the road between going into too much detail and not explaining at all.

Gradually you lose your friends and become less and less keen to try anything new.

Losses

All these things are losses. You may lose friends, self-esteem, your job and your function and roles in life. Personal relationships, your fitness and hobbies may become difficult. Even the ability to relax or sleep comfortably may be affected. If you have suffered these kinds of losses then depression is a very common result. It is one of the three Ds of chronic pain, drugs, disability and depression.

I know this all sounds bad, like there is no hope of getting back to some kind of normality. However, you can control some of these problems and have a much more satisfying life than you might otherwise have.

The management of chronic pain is a complex matter and we need to address many aspects. This book looks at the planning and control of activities when you have a pain problem.

My aim is to give you a clear strategy for managing your pain which suits you best and allows you to get the best out of your life.

Chronic Pain and Activity

Chronic pain always changes what you do and the ways you do it. This varies from small alterations to very great changes in the way you live your life.

In our pain management programmes we always asked what activities were affected by the pain and we always got a long list. Here are some of the examples:

- Loss of work or limited ability to work

- "I can't walk any distance at all nowadays"

- Unable to spend long periods in a car, restricting visits to friends or family who live any distance away

- Withdrawal from social contact - "I can't go dancing with my husband any more"

- Taking lots of medication, with all the side effects

• "I just can't get a good night's sleep"

• Lowering of mood, depression and anxiety

• Increased smoking or drinking alcohol

• Severe reduction or loss of sexual activity

• More arguments and conflicts within the family

• "I can't do normal housework or fix anything useful in the home"

• "I can't pursue my normal hobbies and interests"

• Unwilling to try new things or go to visit people

• "I can't do anything off the cuff" - a need to plan everything carefully

• Pushing to complete activities, then having to rest or lie down.

Once these changes have been going for a while they easily become habits. Many people admit to most of the above losses which have forced them to adapt to a large number of changes. This is challenging.

The control chronic pain exerts over someone's life can become very frustrating. Many people express feelings of hopelessness. This can interfere with efforts to improve your situation.

Rest

Isn't rest a good thing for an injury?

This is a reasonable thing to think but the trouble is, it can lead to severe problems if you take it too seriously. Or keep it up for too long. **There is no good evidence that rest is an effective treatment for low back pain for example**.

If you have severe pain, then it is sensible to "rest" until the pain subsides to a reasonable level. Otherwise the scientific evidence strongly supports activity as a good management strategy for pain.

What are the consequences of resting a lot for pain? I'm afraid this can make things worse. As you do less and less your body becomes weaker and stiffer very quickly.

If you rest completely, i.e. in bed, you can lose 3% of your muscle power every day. This means you get out of physical condition for normal life very quickly. As you do less and lose fitness, you become able to do less and get trapped in a vicious circle.

The psychological consequences, such as loss of confidence, can be just as disabling. You can become isolated from friends and colleagues and suffer depression due to inability to do normal things. Friction in or breakdown of personal relationships is common.

And the good news?

Well, the good news is you can do something about it. Don't get the idea that everything can be wonderful and you can go back to doing what you could in the past.

You are likely to continue to have some problems with your pain, because if the solution was easy you would have already improved.

You can try and stop the decline in your physical abilities and have a more satisfying life. By doing more of the activities you want more of the time. This can have lots of positive knock-on effects on your body, your mind and your personal relationships.

Let's move on to looking at what happens to the body when we don't use it.

The Effects of Inactivity

Our bodies have an amazing ability to adapt to the challenges we set them. If we need to lift heavy weights in a job or in the gym, it responds by quickly building muscle size and strength. If we need to run distances it responds by losing weight and building better blood supplies to our heart and legs.

But if a demand on our body stops occurring, then it lets the extras go very quickly. Why maintain large muscle bulk if it is never used? Since it's no longer required, the body loses much of the bulk to adapt to the new situation.

This same process occurs if we stop doing normal activities. The loss of activity impacts on a large number of body systems, decreasing their ability to function well. If we are only living in the kitchen, why keep up the mansion?

Use it or lose it. Everyone says this at some time. In this context it really does have an important message. If we don't use our body systems they will become less and less able to do the jobs we want them to do.

Let's look at the effects of inactivity on our body systems, one by one.

Bone

Our skeleton is not a fixed thing like the steel inside a concrete building. Imagine you live in a brick house. Every year you pay a bricklayer to take out 15% of the bricks and replace them with new ones. After six or seven years it's still the same house. But all the bricks are different.

Our bones are like that. They are always changing, losing calcium and then building it up again. They are active tissues, not just a static support. If we put large loads on our bodies, our bones respond by becoming denser and stronger.

So if we take to bed and rest, we start to lose the calcium in our bones as they respond to our reduced need for activity. We can lose 40% of the calcium in our bones if we are on bed rest for six months.

Prolonged and strict resting can lead to significant loss of bone mass which can increase the risk of fracture under load.

Joints

Our joints are built to move. That's what they're for and they don't take kindly to being still for long periods. We have all stretched out our knees after having them cramped up in the back of a car for too long. I remember it being painful and being unable to walk properly for a short while.

A lack of activity over a long time can increase joint stiffness as the fibrous surrounds of the joint tighten to some degree. Loss of muscle power around the joint can make them less stable. This can reduce the control of the joint and increase the chance of injury.

Muscles and Tendons

About 30% of our body weight is muscle which indicates its importance. It is expensive to make and maintain muscle so the body only does it if it's really needed.

After 24 hours bed rest we lose 3% of our muscle strength, so you can see that after a week or so with 'flu you will be a lot weaker. No wonder you feel wobbly when you get up and about again.

Inactivity leads to a loss of muscle bulk and strength, with loss of flexibility, the ability to stretch. Long term rest can lead to muscles becoming more fibrous and resistant to stretch.

The Cardiovascular System

This includes the heart, lungs and blood vessels around the body. Though it is less obvious, our system for pumping oxygenated blood around the body can be fitter or less fit.

Our hearts are muscles as well. A different kind of muscle to the regular or skeletal muscles of our arms and legs but a muscle all the same.

Like all muscles, the heart responds to exercise. If exercised, it becomes larger and fitter, pumping more blood with less effort. If rested it becomes smaller and less able at pumping blood.

To be active our cardiovascular system should respond to us starting to do something. We need increased supplies of blood and oxygen to our muscles when we do an activity. Our heart can provide this if it is fit enough.

If we are unfit it is difficult for our heart, lungs and blood vessels to provide the oxygenated blood required quickly enough. This will limit what we can do.

Inactivity can lead to a smaller heart, fatty deposits in the heart and coronary vessels, increased blood pressure and smaller red blood cells.

All this can result in a system that's unfit for duty.

The Brain

Circulation and oxygenation of the brain may reduce, leading to a feeling of tiredness and doziness. Inactivity is depressing, tends to make us feel more tired and less able to cope with stress. It may also lead to depression due to the loss of the things we used to do.

It would be unfortunate to have all these problems. But it is likely that anyone who has been inactive for a sustained period would have some or most on this list.

Pain may not be the initial cause of these many problems. Loss of activity due to pain may be the cause. Fortunately we can reverse loss of activity and improve our ability to get things done.

Sport and Pacing

Pacing is not only good for dealing with pain problems, but an essential and everyday part of athletic training. Well, of successful athletic training anyhow.

Ask yourself - "Does world record holding sprinter Usain Bolt just turn up at the Olympic 100 metre sprint and have a go?" or "When he's training does he just run round a bit and do a few sprints?"

Of course not. If we had Usain's training schedule in front of us I'm sure we'd be looking at pages and pages of figures. Those figures would show how much he was to do of what activity, how much resistance there was to be and how often he was to do it. He increases the stresses he puts on his body tissues very precisely until he gets to the Olympic 100 metre final. Then he can go all out to win and break the world record.

Usain's a fit guy, so why mess about with all this precise control of what he's doing every day?

Because we all have body tissues which respond the same way to use. If underused they lose some of their ability and if they overused they can suffer damage and may give pain.

Usain has to follow this careful and disciplined climb to peak condition and fitness. If he did not, his performance could not be at peak level. And the forces he puts on his tissues when he sprints hard could easily cause a hamstring tear or a tendon rupture.

Sports training is also very specific. If you're fit for one sport you're not fit for another. And participating in a sport you're not trained for puts you at risk of injury no matter how fit you are for another sport.

Now you've seen the things that can go wrong and we've talked about body tissues and how much stress to put on them for how long. That leads us easily on to tissue tolerances, a key idea you need to get straight.

5

The Body and Its Tissues

What Our Bodies Have To Cope With

THE BODY IS an amazing machine. If we're lucky it functions for many, many years without complaint, carrying us around as we do what we want.

But it's not invincible.

We know our bones can break if we fall from a height or get hit by a car, and that bullets are bad for us. But we can disturb the smooth working of the body in more subtle ways.

Our body tissues are all designed to do certain jobs: to support weight; to contract; to carry blood; to move. But like a machine's parts, the body has performance limits. Our limits of what the body can do vary all the time with our age, fitness, pain problems, recent training and other factors.

We can push our luck in all sorts of ways. Lift something way too heavy or workout hard in the gym when we haven't been for three months, cycle 20 miles when we normally do two or three miles.

Dig the whole vegetable garden in one go or clean the house from top to bottom.

This has effects on the tissues and tests their tolerances.

Tissue Tolerances

I know that tissue tolerances sounds a bit biological for most people but stick with me. The idea of our body parts having a limit for physical stresses is an important one. It can help you see why doing what you do is giving you the problems you have. It could even reassure you why you are trying that funny Pacing System thing at all.

At all stages of our lives the tissues of our bodies have a specific tolerance for physical stresses. This means our muscles, tendons or bones will take a certain amount of use or abuse from us before they complain.

If we are young then overdoing an activity will lead to a bit of stiffness the next day. If we are older it can lead to us feeling like a crock for several days and being less keen to do it again.

We're all superbly designed to do our daily activities so we can achieve the things we want to or have to do.

Our body tissues cope with the demands of moving us about and any jobs we must do. We don't usually think about it at all, we just get on with the things we are doing.

Until, that is, suddenly we have to do something different, something heavier or for a much longer period of time. Then we notice. Even then, it may not matter much, just a feeling of muscle strain or an ache in a joint which settles in hours or days.

When I was 20 I found an American muscle magazine in a shop. I had never seen bodies like that! I decided I could do with a bit more muscle so went to a local gym and did the beginner's workout from the magazine.

The next day I couldn't move! It was three days before I could get dressed in the normal way.

That event had a profound effect on my thoughts and behaviour. First I just avoided the gym. If it was so painful it was obviously unsafe! Then I got over this and did it better, with some success.

So what went wrong?

I was a skinny guy with long arms and legs and who had not done much hard physical work in my life up until then. My tissues were just not prepared for the forces I suddenly put on them.

Sport and Tissue Tolerances

Although work practices and poor posture can strain our tissues, it is in sport that we treat our bodies most badly.

Millions of people take up running, or gym workouts, or any sport, with little or no preparation. Many find the unpleasant results after the first try are enough to stop the activity right away. Others push themselves to perform better and better and overstep the tolerances of their tissues.

Training for sports is very specific. This means the body needs to train for the particular sport performance chosen. Whilst it's good to be fit and be able to run a distance, this won't help you much to play football or to swim far.

We pay too little attention to preparing our bodies for the requirements of the sport or activity we have chosen. Season after season of sport can take its toll on our joints and other tissues, storing up problems for later. Arthritis in our joints is a common consequence of treating our bodies badly such as in sport.

Olympians Do It

Athletes pace. The fittest and strongest people on earth do this because they know that any other strategy will fail. Push hard all the time and you will overtrain or injure yourself. Train as you feel and you'll never get to that peak condition.

Using pacing and sports strategies such as periodic training, you have a chance of getting into your best shape at the right time.

It's the same with any kind of pain problem. You can choose to push yourself for something important if you wish. A day out with the grandchildren may be more important than the extra pain you will suffer for a few days. That might make good sense to you. You accept the increased pain and decreased ability for a few days. The only risk here is if you do that often you may become more disabled with time. This might not happen, but it's worth thinking about.

Exercise and Micro-Trauma

When we exercise, we cause what we call micro-trauma to the muscles concerned. This microscopic muscle damage is good, as it forces our muscles to repair, which they do by getting bigger and stronger. Tendons and ligaments can also build up a tolerance to increased activity with training.

This is fine if you don’t overdo it like I did.

I caused myself so much micro-trauma that it wasn’t micro any more! The normal process of inflammation occurred but at a much higher level than I'd anticipated. This gave me a high level of pain for a few days.

I had overstepped the tolerance of my tissues to physical stress, so I paid for it.

You can see people pushing their luck all the time. Spring comes along and we gardeners start mowing, digging and bending over a lot. This leads to a minor epidemic of soft-tissue injuries and overstrains. Which makes physiotherapists and osteopaths very happy!

When we try and take up a new activity or sport we often find that the first effort gives us significant problems. Many people give up at that point, not expecting a severe reaction.

If you overstep your tissue tolerances you will pay too. You may already have paid, and often, if you are reading this.

Tissue Tolerances and Pain Problems

What I have just covered applies to "normal" people, by which I mean people with no musculo-skeletal problems. It applies just as much to the greatest Olympic athlete as it does to the most dedicated couch potato.

But the effects of overdoing tissue tolerances

become so much more serious when we aren't "normal" people. When we, including me, have a pain problem of some kind.

It can cripple you for a while. It can make you more and more disabled with time so you do less and less. It can make you depressed and make your life so much less satisfying than you had ever expected.

Having a pain problem really brings overdoing into focus. And the reason it's so important is not just due to the tissue tolerance stuff we have just talked about. It's also due to the way the nervous system works in pain problems.

6

THE BOOM & BUST ACTIVITY CYCLE

Stuck In A Cycle

OK, SO YOU wake up one morning and the pain doesn't feel so bad. What happens next?

You think "Wow, it's finally settling down! Now I can get on with all the things I have been putting off. The hall needs decorating and I need some new clothes from the town. I've not seen my friends for a drink for ages and the family deserve a nice meal cooked for them. Let's go for it!"

What happens next?

Full of enthusiasm, you get going on the day's jobs and to start with things go well. You notice some increase in your pain but you think that's ok and move on to the next chore.

After a while you feel the pain more severely and begin to slow down your headlong rush to get things done.

At some later time the pain becomes severe enough to stop you in your tracks and you have to leave any outstanding activities and rest. But to your horror, the pain does not then begin to settle and becomes steadily worse.

What happens next?

The pain builds up to a severe level, completely disabling you and stopping all but the most essential activities. You lie down to rest and find sleep difficult or impossible.

You take the highest permitted (or even higher - not recommended) doses of your pain medication. Or you may resort to drugs or alcohol. The next few days or weeks are hell, as the pain remains at a severe level and you are able to do very little.

What effect does this have on you?

Resting for a long time with pain is a depressing experience and feels like a waste of your life. Severe pain is a punishing experience and makes you uncertain about repeating what caused the problem.

However, resting does help the pain to some extent so you may feel that rest is one of the right ways to manage your pain.

This is one of the main parts of this book. It's vital to understand the over and under-activity cycle if you are to tackle your pain problems.

When we want to do something, we just want to get it done. We rarely think about how we are going to do it, we usually just concentrate on getting it completed. This is often fine until we take on too much or have a pain condition.

Overuse injuries are common. Tennis elbow, shin splints, back problems and shoulder tendon pains are all examples. We are careless and don't take care of our body tissues while we do repetitive or forceful movements in our jobs or hobbies.

The Over-Activity Cycle

This is a common habit we all share at one time or another. We push ourselves to complete the window cleaning, the digging of the vegetable plot or the painting of the house. These are only three of many possible examples. I'm sure you can come up with some which are special to you.

A few days of pain or strain may be the only consequences of overdoing a particular activity. But if an activity is overdone often enough it can lead to a longer lasting problem as the pain comes on sooner and sooner in the job.

The pain still goes away though. At least at first. Then comes the time when you have to do the same job again and the pain stops you completing it but this time it doesn't go away. It settles to some degree but remains at a low level. If you try the job again at any time the pain increases so fast that you have to stop pretty quickly.

You now have an overuse problem. This will limit your ability to do the job in future and perhaps some related activities. It is difficult to fix this kind of problem once the pain has set in.

This over-activity cycle is also common in sport.

So Why Is The Boom and Bust Activity Cycle Such A Bad Thing?

Well, I'm sure you've got the hang of some of the reasons by now. If you push yourself hard you will suffer a lot of pain afterwards and this has effects.

1. You will be less keen to do the activity again so you avoid it in the future and are able gradually to do less and less.

2. You may get frustrated and depressed in the painful period when you are forced to rest.

3. The pain forces you to rest which makes you less fit and less able to do things in the future.

4. Your pain may worsen even though you are not doing much and certainly less than you were a year or two previously.

There's the rub. If you get stuck in this over/underactivity cycle your pain may become worse and your physical ability reduce over time.

Frankly, you are becoming steadily more disabled, and who wants that? Keep going in this cycle and the results are going to be very depressing.

Overdoing

Overdoing is the most common response to a challenging pain problem. Or a challenging goal.

But what is overdoing? It doesn't matter whether you feel you should be able to do something easily. Or if you could always do the same activity in the past. Having a severe pain reaction and coming to a stop, that makes it overdoing for me.

You’re trying to get things done and pushing yourself to complete what you have planned. At some point you're forced to stop as your pain has become significantly worse and then you're stuck. That's what overdoing is. And overdoing always leads to under-doing, in other words resting.

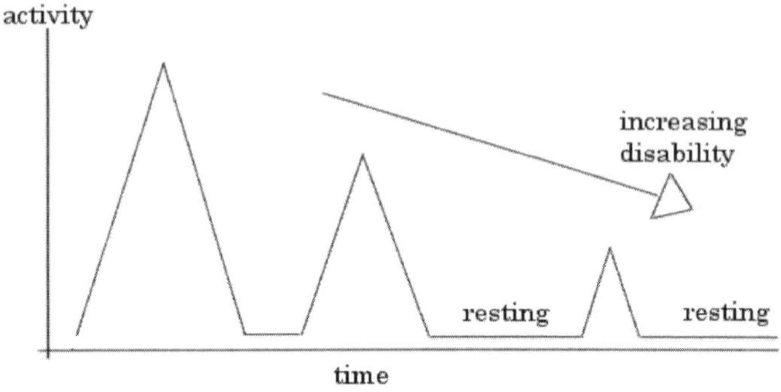

This is what the Boom and Bust activity cycle looks like as a diagram. The peaks show the levels of activity. As you can see, after the high peaks periods of forced inactivity follow.

With time, the peaks you can achieve get lower (you can do less and less) and the periods of inactivity get longer. This means that your disability is getting gradually worse.

This diagram is just an illustration and in reality the graph will be a lot more irregular, drawn out and untidy. But it gives the impression I want to get across to you.

Is that it then? Unfortunately not.

When you push yourself your pain gets gradually worse and worse until it forces you to lie down or to back off your activity. Then the pain remains at a high level for a day or two, allowing you to do very little during this time.

And that's depressing. And a waste of time. And frustrating.

When the pain settles again what happens? Do we learn from our previous experiences and change the way we do things?

Fat chance!

The next time we feel OK we do it all over again.

We do not seem to learn from our mistakes. Yes, I have been the same, until I understood this and even then it took someone else to push me into doing it right eventually. It's a natural thing just to have a go at things, and pacing is a very unnatural concept.

Most people do understand that this pattern is self-defeating but seem unable to break out of it on their own. They know it's important to be active and keep on with normal life as much as possible.

Avoiding

Avoiding is also known as under-doing.

"So how long on average do you spend lying down over a 24 hour period then?" I asked the 22 year old young man who had attended for assessment with the pain management team.

“Oh about 23 hours out of 24” He replied. He and his girlfriend stayed on the bed all day. I can’t remember if she had a back problem too… They bought in food and ate it lying down. They watched TV most of the time. They only got up to go to the toilet or fetch something to eat or drink.

This was I admit an extreme case of avoidance of normal activity, even of standing up and walking about. But it shows how far into a hole some people can get, far enough so they can’t dig themselves out.

Think back to the chapter on chronic pain. If you have not addressed the hurt and harm idea and still have a strong fear of further injury, it might seem reasonable to spend all day in bed.

Overdoing always leads to this second half of the cycle - under-doing or avoiding. If one activity, or many activities, are painful then one way of managing them is to avoid them altogether.

Yet this approach can have its problems just like overdoing.

If you start avoiding a particularly difficult activity you may feel this is a reasonable approach, and indeed it may be. But it is easy for this approach to creep up on you and suddenly you find yourself avoiding a whole stack of activities.

In fact you can wake up one morning and realise that you are doing very little every day. Like the young guy above, although I hope not so dramatically.

Can you see the possible patterns? People vary a lot in how they behave in response to chronic pain problems. Some overdo activities all the time and find themselves constantly fighting against pain flare-ups.

Others avoid almost all activities and spend most of the day and night lying down. Most common is a mix of the two. **People with chronic pain are not lazy and overdoing is more common than avoiding**.

Anxiety about the pain is brought on by activities due to the fear of further injury. This leads to avoidance until a job comes up which you have to do. Or the pain settles steadily and makes you think you can go for it again.

Back into the cycle!

Some people just keep on going round and round as if they've got stuck. And stuck is the best way of thinking about it. Something new has to happen before this can change.

7

ARE YOU SUSCEPTIBLE?

Personality Matters

THE PEOPLE MOST likely to fall into this cycle are ironically the same people who find it the hardest to apply the solution.

1. You like to get things done

Can you hear yourself saying “If a job's worth doing it's worth doing well” and “Don't start something you don't mean to finish”?

You may or may not be a perfectionist, but doing the job well means a lot to you and how you feel about yourself. You may see it as a failure if you do not reach the goal you have set yourself in terms of either time or quality.

It may seem like the Eleventh Commandment to continue a task until complete, whatever it costs in pain or loss of activity. Perhaps it is something you learned as a young person from those around you and have carried with you throughout life.

Any other way of doing things seems to be very much second best so this kind of approach to activities is difficult to alter.

2. You're competitive

If you push yourself to achieve from an internal sense of competition, or to show others you can still cut it, you are likely to overdo madly.

“I won't let it beat me” is a common quote from your sort of personality. It is as though the pain is a separate person and must not be allowed to dominate. So you push hard and continue to do the things you want or have to do, and to hell with the pain.

It's not gonna win, no sir! But it’s a sneaky enemy and creeps up on you. Changing this point of view is not going to be easy.

3. “My back's damaged and fragile”

Now this thought is going to lead to problems.

If your main worry is the damage and injury which is continuing in your back then you’ll likely do the opposite of overdoing. This is avoiding. That makes sense after all doesn't it? If I am damaging myself by an activity, it's surely right to stop doing it.

One of my patients said to my colleague the clinical psychologist “My back is like a stack of digestive biscuits”. If you think your back’s fragile and crumbling, how likely are you to take the advice of the nice physiotherapist to do this or that exercise? Not very. Before he can think about increasing his activities he needs to address his beliefs about his back.

The problem comes when you suddenly notice you are avoiding most or all activities and doing very little.

How did that happen? Trying to reverse this trend will make you feel anxious as you increase your activities and confront your worries. This is known as fear-avoidance and is important in understanding how people can become disabled.

Fear-Avoidance

In fear-avoidance, fear of what has happened or what might happen is the central idea. When an injury or pain occurs, we all have an emotional response to it. We all think something about it, and we all have feelings about what is going on.

How we react emotionally to our pain and injury problem has profound effects on how or even whether we recover well.

Let's look at what can happen. Confrontation and avoidance are the two extreme reactions to this fear of activity.

Confrontation

You confront pain when you have little fear of what is going on. So you gradually increase your activity levels until you get back to normal. Even though you get some increases in pain as you do more, you do not worry about this and keep going. The problem settles and you get back to normal life.

Avoidance

Avoidance has much more potential for severe problems. Here you have high levels of fear about what is going on in your back and make decisions about your activity based on this fear.

You interpret internal body sensations negatively. You think there's something wrong or damaged and suffer from a lowered mood and feel anxious. This leads to:

• The adoption of avoidance behaviour, which causes you to do less as you avoid normal activity.

• You become over-aware of feelings coming in from your body and the information you may read or get from others. You interpret this information negatively in terms of your recovery.

• You become over-reactive. Your system reacts badly to normal postures and activity, giving you pain when it used not to.

• You become de-conditioned, weaker and do less as you become more guarded and more careful with movement.

To manage fear-avoidance I have tried to carefully explain what is going on. You will need to address your specific fears about what's going on in your back or other areas. You can then progress by gradual exposure to your fears without triggering the unpleasant reaction.

Only when you start to do something you fear without severe consequences can you build confidence and move forward.

8

How to Pace

Doing It

HERE'S WHERE WE get to actually doing it. We've had all the theory, it's time to get on and pace. As with any skill, it's important to have a go, make mistakes, learn and move forward. Appendix 4 has "My Pacing Worksheet" if you want to fill in the blanks as you go along.

1. Choose an activity you typically overdo and suffer pain afterwards. You will know what activity tends to make you worse and the one you do most often. Pick your worst habit, the one you push at most, as this will give you the greatest benefit if you can get it under control. Other difficulties may melt away if you control the big one. It could be ironing, hoovering or something like sitting. That's an activity too.

2. Perform this activity until your pain STARTS to worsen. DO NOT go on as far as you can manage. It's very important you don't try and find out how much you can do, in other words the maximum. You are trying to find the point where your pain is beginning to be affected by the activity but does not stir it up greatly. Then STOP!

3. Record this length of time. Write it down, how long you managed the activity in minutes. Or the number of times you did something. Whatever you do, it's important to get a precise measurement so you can work with it.

4. Repeat stages 2 and 3 a few times, at intervals. It's important to do the measurement a few times. You could take a measurement when you were having much more or much less pain than normal and this would mess up the calculations. A few measurements smoothe out any likely errors here.

5. Take an average of your readings. Easy enough. Add up all the minutes and divide them by the number of readings you have taken. Make sure you record this number.

6. Take 20% off your average. There's no particular magic or scientific foundation to taking 20% off. It's just something that seems to work. You are taking 20% off the average figure for the activity which does not aggravate your pain significantly. This should ensure it's low enough for you to achieve it regularly and not have a pain problem afterwards. Record this number too.

7. Use this figure as the amount of time you do

the activity. This is the start of the disciplined bit. You need to accept that the time you have worked out is one you can accept. You have to believe it's ok to do the activity for ONLY this amount of time. For a while anyhow.

8. Stick to this figure and DO NOT go over it. No excuses. Yes it's that rigid! For now you have to stick to the time you have worked out. Otherwise you won't regain control of your pain and your life. Once you have learned the ropes you can be more flexible. But for now, stick absolutely to your time. Use a kitchen timer or the timer on a smartphone to alert you. It's very easy to go over time without thinking. No "Well I was almost finished so I thought I'd just complete it…".

9. Leave at least twice your pacing time between paced sessions. There's no real science behind this timing either! It's just something I consider is the minimum to allow your pain levels to subside. You could choose to leave much longer between your sessions of activity if you want.

10. Perform a suitable number of repetitions but do not necessarily try to complete the activity. I can't tell how many times you should do your paced sessions in one go. Just don't try and do as many as you can. Or try and achieve more than you usually can. And the aim is not to complete the task. It's to do an amount of activity without provoking your pain significantly. So don't try and finish the job. Just stop when you think you should.

11. When you do it well, reward yourself. If you succeed at this difficult task then it's important to recognise this. Rewarding yourself with something will make it just a little bit easier to continue doing something. Especially something you'd rather not be doing. See "Changing Behaviour" for more on this.

12. When you've done this for a while and you can do your pacing time easily, decide to increase your quota. If it's going well you will have done your paced activity several times without any real effects in terms of pain. Keep on with this controlled plan until you're sure that you can easily manage the time without any problems. Now it's time to increase your quota time, not just to see how much you can do.

13. Increase the quota by a planned amount, not more than 10% of the total. Time to increase your quota. It's vital to decide this before you start the activity again rather than just have a go and see how much you can do. Increasing by 10% is a good start as this still keeps you under your initial measurement time for the moment.

14. Use this increased amount as your new

quota. You know what to do by now. Use the new quota time to control your activity. Stick to the time no matter how inconvenient or stupid it may seem. It's the route towards the control you are seeking.

15. Continue the process until you feel you can do things as you wish or any more increases would worsen your pain. You may meet a plateau where you feel you can't go any further without problems. You may have to accept this. With time you can stop your deterioration in ability and turn it around.

16. "Internalise" your ability to pace. This means your brain understands how to pace and tells you when you have done enough. And you take notice. This allows you to be free of a clock or timer. Now you can pace naturally without thinking.

That's all there is to it! It's very simple in theory, the hard part is to make yourself stick to the quota you have set. That's hard. See "The 5 Principles of Pacing" and "The 6 Traps" to explain more why you are doing it this way. And how to avoid setbacks which can be discouraging.

9

The 5 Principles of Pacing

Applying What You Have Learned

WELL DONE! YOU'VE stuck with all the initial stuff about pain, about behaviour and the consequences. Now it's time to get to the meat of what we are talking about. To walk the walk.

The whole idea of this book is to apply the principles to doing things in normal life. If you change the way you do things and find it useful, I will have achieved my aim.

Once you have realised you are in the unhelpful cycle of overactivity and underactivity, you can start to work at it. The aim is to increase the level of your activities without stirring up your pain badly. That way you can begin to get back to your normal activities.

Being realistic is important. There may be some activities you used to do which you are never going to be able to perform again. Part of the process is to generate alternatives, new ideas which can take you forward. But people can achieve surprising things with time. Just don't start off with a hugely ambitious goal.

Begin pacing with an activity you want to perform but find difficult. Do it for just one activity to start with to measure the results and get the idea clear in your head.

Pacing is a simple idea but it is not easy to implement. There are traps out there and you can fall into them. In the next chapter I will try and point out as many of them to you as I can, so you can adopt pacing successfully.

Let's get on to the detail.

Principle One

In pacing, it's your brain which makes the decisions about your activity, NOT your pain

When Pain's In Control - "Pain Dependent Activity"

Remember what you have just read in the preceding few pages about doing activities under the control of your pain. Pain has been the dictator, telling you to start or stop an activity.

You have been the unhappy slave to your pain, and we call this pain-dependent activity or exercise. This means that your activity depends on the state of your pain at the time. If you are in a good phase, you do it. If you are in a bad one you stop. Pain is the master. It has all the disadvantages previously discussed.

When You're In Control - "Time-Dependent Activity"

"What's that?" I hear you say. Well, hang on and I'll explain.

Normally we keep going with an activity until it's finished, we're bored or it hurts. Then we stop. This attitude is fine when we do not have a pain or other health problem but becomes a problem when we do.

To avoid the Boom and Bust Cycle we need another way of doing things.

Setting times for the things you do and sticking to those times is the key to pacing.

Simple? Yes. Difficult? Yes!

Your mind still thinks you're 21 and have the body to match. It thinks you are as you were, as you remember yourself in the past and as you think you should be.

Getting over this and understanding you are not as you were is very hard, but you will not be able to move forward and pace successfully unless you do. Remember, this is particularly hard for competitive and "I like to get things done" people.

What's the alternative? You could go on as you were. But by buying this book you have shown you are not satisfied with some aspects of your life and want to change them.

Think about my suggestions as an experiment which you can try for a while and see how it goes. If it goes well, great! If not so well, you have not lost anything but a little time.

Principle Two

When you do well and succeed at your pacing task, reward yourself!

It can't all be bad can it? There's got to be some pleasure, surely?

When you do well, reward yourself! This is based on a psychological principle - "Any behaviour followed by a reward is more likely to be repeated".

Think carefully about that. If you want a child to be good, a dog to come back to you or a builder to do a good job on your house extension, you need to use a reward. We do this all the time.

This principle holds for us all, child or adult alike. It also works well for your dog, though not necessarily so well with your cat.

And you do need help to keep up pacing. After you have successfully paced an activity you should reward yourself. If you stopped yourself overdoing and didn't suffer unduly after, you’ve done amazingly well. Give yourself a reward!

Examples of rewards are a cup of tea and a biscuit, a glass of wine, a walk in the sun, buying a paper or magazine or watching a programme on the TV. You will have some you particularly like, so use them!

It's important that you take your rewards straight after the successful pacing attempt. You must be able to give yourself the reward, i.e. you do not have to rely on someone else. And don't give yourself the reward before the job is done.

Would you pay the builder for your new extension up front at the start? Why not? Because you may get rather slow service or, if you are unlucky, no service at all.

One more thing. Don't reward yourself if you don't do well! Save your rewards until you succeed next time. No, don't punish yourself. You have enough pain as it is and punishment is much less successful than reward for getting someone to do something.

Principle Three

Measure the time or activity precisely, and don't just guess

So how did John in Chapter 1 get an accurate measurement of his easy tolerance for his particular activity? He took several measurements and averaged them out. One measurement might have happened to occur at a particularly bad or good time for John.

Let's say John takes several measurements of how long he can easily mow the grass. We get times of 25 minutes, 35 minutes, 20 minutes and 40 minutes (can you see I'm making this easy for myself?!). Now we have to do a bit of Math and this should not tax anyone's ability. The average is 30 minutes.

Next step is to reduce this by an amount which will allow John to mow for a length of time which will not bring on his back pain significantly.

There is no magic answer here but routinely we take 20% of this figure. That's 24 minutes because I've done this calculation before! So, what do we do with this figure of 24 minutes?

The key point here is to work out an exact amount of time or number of repetitions to do something. Don't rely on how you feel.

This leads to my fourth principle.

Principle Four

When you've worked out your quota, never go over it

Quotas and stopping when you should

Yes, 24 minutes is John's quota. A quota is an amount which you are not meant to exceed.

Once you have figured out this amount it is vital not to go over it.

So John gets a timer or uses his watch and starts to mow the grass. When he gets to 24 minutes he stops and walks away from the mower.

"What? Stop a quarter way through?", you say, "I can't do that!"

- Yes, I know it's difficult.
- Yes, I know it'll take too long
- Yes, I know you like/must/have to keep going

until the task is done

• Yes I know you’ve always done it that way

• Yes, I know you don’t feel you can change at your stage in life.

Remember, this is an experiment in how you can change things because your present behaviour is giving you problems.

Pacing will allow you to complete what you want to do, and not have the awful consequences after. Or it will allow you to start something again, something you have wanted to do but were afraid of the effects.

“What”, I hear you ask, “do I do after the 24 minutes is up and I have stopped the task, and when can I get started again?”

The intervals between your activity do not have to be resting as such. You don't need to go and lie down, the time should be just not doing that particular task. You could have two or three jobs on the go and could do small amounts of each.

Doing something similar in physical terms would not make much sense either. You need to choose something different, involving perhaps a different position. When you feel you have had enough "rest" you can go back and do another 24 minutes.

What, you say you are already doing things this way?

I don't think so. With respect, you may be pacing, but it is much more likely you are doing an activity for a time until your pain tells you there's a problem. Then you stop.

You may not push madly into the pain but you are still stopping too late to gain real control over your pain.

So what's the end result, the perfect technique? That's when you estimate your pacing times correctly and stick to them. With suitable rests between periods of activity. That way you will complete the task you wanted to do and not suffer a significant increase in your pain for a significant length of time.

Success!

You've done it and not disabled yourself. Don't forget to reward yourself now.

TIP

Don't feel you have to get the task done in one day. You will have to work out how many paced sessions you can do without a problem.

TIP

Say this to yourself when you tempted to push. "I am making myself more disabled". This idea may help you stick to your plan.

Principle Five

Always decide how much to increase your quota BEFORE you start

If you get going with the activity and try and work out how much more you can manage while you're doing it you are very likely to overdo it.

When you have discovered how much is too much it will be too late.

Take a sensible amount of increase which does not represent a large proportion of the quota amount and add it to your quota. Done! That's your new quota and you do not need my reminder to stick to it.....do you?

10% is a sensible level to increase to start with, though you may prefer larger or smaller increases for your particular tasks.

The good news is that in some cases you can continue increasing your quotas. Eventually they might reach what for you might be reasonable times. Then you will be doing the maximum you sensibly can for the problems you have.

10

SUCCEED WITH PACING

Making Success Easy

PACING IS A simple concept. Your brain decides now much activity you do rather than the feelings which come in from your body.

Is it easy? No chance! If you really need to pace you will really find it difficult. So how can you make it easier?

Taking it easy – how to help yourself succeed

Think of pacing as an experiment, to try for a while and see how it goes. If you test it and find it useful you will be convinced.

Don't expect to see changes too soon. It takes time for changes to occur in a situation which has lasted a long time. Why would it change that quickly?

Think of all the times you spend doing very little because your pain is much worse. How much do you get done then? If you pace you may get much more done overall due to less wasted time recovering from episodes of overdoing.

You wouldn't expect to get a big job done in one hour or one day, so why do other jobs have to be completed in one go?

You Can Change. Recognise that the way you behave is not fixed, it's just something you have learned as a child or young person, and you can change that.

Decide what your choice is going to be, for it is a choice you have to make. Do you go on following the old ways or try something new which just might help?

Pick Winners. When you start to pace, choose your worst pain-pushing habit first. This way you will get a success at the outset. Let's say you always go mad with the housework or the lawn-mowing. Work on those activities as they are likely to have the greatest effect on your pain and ability.

Other People can get in the way. Sometimes other people get in the way. Often they don't mean to and they do it out of the best of motives, but they can still stop you pacing correctly or trying new activities. You need to recognise this and take steps to fix the problem.

"No, no, don't do that, you know what happened last time, you were laid up for a week. Let me do it!"

Did you relate to that? Is it something your nearest and dearest has said to you, with an air of exasperation, as you try to do something? How are you going to keep the domestic peace and still make progress?

A bit of communication and explanation is good here to reassure the anxious person that it is ok for you to do these things. That's all that's usually needed.

Research has shown that some people with pain have very helpful spouses and families, who do almost everything for the pain sufferer. Unfortunately these people are more disabled than people who have to manage more on their own.

So it's good that you explain to your significant others and get them to appreciate that you need to be allowed to do more physically. And it won't do you any harm or result in days of severe pain increase. If you pace, that is...

"Get on with it, you can't leave it like that, or I'll have to do it. You are so slow, I think you're getting lazy. And there's still the bathroom and the garage"

This is a different one. The speaker is not happy here and blaming the sufferer for performing below expectations. The sufferer is not coming up to their standards and perhaps doing jobs in a paced way is not acceptable due to the increased time it takes.

Communication and assertiveness are again the keys to resolving these situations. Don't get the idea they always work! But they have a much greater chance of working than any other strategy.

Assertiveness is a big subject and I will be covering that and communication in another book in the series.

Getting It Right

What should you notice when you get pacing right?

1. Those good and bad days should be less noticeable and you should have more reasonable days.

2. Pushing yourself may well have been followed by bad days in the past but now these can be cut out, smoothing out the ups and downs in both your activity and your pain.

3. On good days you decide not to do more than normal, just enjoy the better day for your pain.

4. On worse days you do not back off completely and rest, but keep up some level of activity.

Here's an illustration of a paced activity session:

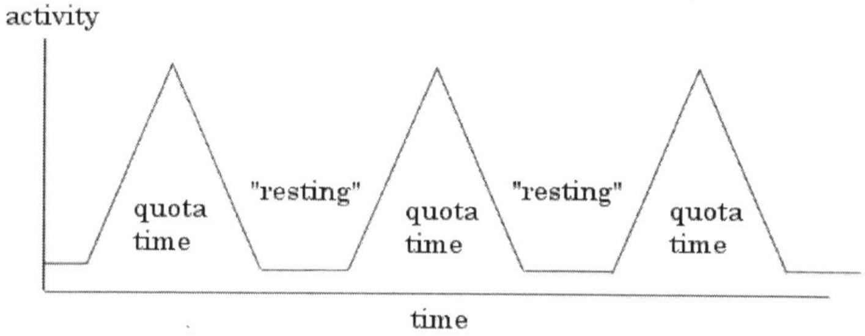

You can see in this diagram that the peaks of activity are all the same, as that is the previously decided paced amount. The "resting" inbetween, which are periods not doing that activity rather than actual rest, are also regular and pre-planned. This way you are in control of your activity and your pain is not.

What you will learn

• The first thing is you CAN be disciplined and stick to your quotas on the good days. You can use your determination in a different way and follow a programme which promises benefits.

• Second, it will dawn on you that you have control over your pain rather than the other way round.

This is vital if you are going to be able to plan your life for yourself and others.

• Thirdly you will realize that even on a bad day you can keep going and complete your quota of activity. This will make you feel more of an achiever, increase your self esteem and make you understand that you can still be active despite the pain.

If you pace yourself successfully it may hurt, but it is not doing you any bodily harm. Remember back to the "Hurt equals Harm" idea in the chapter on pain.

11

THE 6 TRAPS

Overcoming The Obstacles

I'VE LISTENED TO hundreds of people tell me their stories of pain. Always interesting, these stories began to sort themselves in my brain. I started to see patterns which occur again and again. One pattern which stuck out was the way things could go wrong.

In the ocean of pain there are icebergs. You can bump into them hard without knowing they are there. They are the hidden obstacles to progress which can stop you in your tracks.

I've sorted them into six categories for you so you can understand them and see them coming. This will help you to be successful in your pacing attempts.

Trap No.1

"I can't change; I've always done things this way."

This is a common problem. You may be the kind of

person who likes to get things done, who doesn't like messing around.

You say things to yourself such as "If a thing's worth doing it's worth doing well." and "Never leave anything for tomorrow if you can do it today."

This means you have a strong drive to complete activities and do not like the untidiness of leaving things half done. You have learnt this as a child or young person perhaps, with your parents as a likely model.

Remember, finishing off an activity or chore in one go is not the Eleventh Commandment. It is just the way you have done it in the past. Things are different now or you would not be reading this book.

Antidotes to Trap No. 1

• Think of pacing as an experiment which you do for a while until you can decide whether it is going to be useful or not. That way you do not have to commit yourself to something you're not sure of.

• Recognise that you, like any other person, can change if you want.

• Discuss with your significant others whether it is really necessary to get something done perfectly and completely in one go.

• Think "If I continue as I am, I will waste all that time recovering from a severe pain episode. If I pace I will be able to keep going and get more done."

• Think "Why am I making myself more disabled?"

Trap No.2

"If I do anything, it's got to be done properly. If you want something done well, do it yourself."

Yes, you're a perfectionist and do not trust anyone else to come up to your high standards. So delegation is not one of your strong points.

This attitude can, interestingly, have two almost opposite effects:

1. When you do something you do it thoroughly and completely, never considering cutting corners or leaving it undone. This means you always push to complete an activity and accept you will suffer afterwards.

2. You decide that if you cannot do something really well you will not do it at all. So you never start anything important as you cannot be sure you

can do it properly to your satisfaction.

Antidotes to Trap No. 2

• "Pushing through the pain barrier" just doesn't work when you have a pain problem. And it never will. There is no chance of ever getting where you want to be with this technique.

• What does it matter if you accept a lower standard? Think of it as a temporary concession to allow you to move towards your goal.

• If you do not start to do things you will never be able to move forward. Consider doing part of a job and have someone else complete it. This allows you to achieve something and experience success.

Trap No.3

You wake up and you are having a good day

It's ironic I know, but this is one of the most deadly traps, and it can catch you again and again.

You wake up and the pain is not so bad. "Great!", you say, "Now I can really get some stuff done." You severely overdo things, increase your pain and suffer a period of forced inactivity.

Feeling good is a trap because you are tempted just

to get on with things without thinking.

Antidotes to Trap No. 3

• Read, digest and put this book into action!

• If you pace your activity on a good day, you are more likely to have good days following.

• If you push yourself hard on a good day, you are very likely to have one or two bad days following this.

Trap No.4

You fear ongoing damage in your back or other part, so you do less and less with time

When we get a pain it always has some emotional effect on us, however small. When we get a severe pain, or one we interpret as being caused by serious internal damage of some kind, we can be affected by what is called fear-avoidance.

Remember the information on fear-avoidance? This can lead to a person becoming gradually more disabled with time.

There is no future in seriously avoiding activities, as there is no time in the future when this might turn around and improve. You need to confront the pain to some extent.

Antidotes to Trap No. 4

• Chronic pain can remain way after the original injury has healed. The level of pain experienced does not reflect the level or even presence of tissue damage.

• Examine your own attitudes and beliefs to what is going on inside your back. Is there evidence of inflammation, degeneration and damage, or does it just FEEL like there is?

• Realise that rest is not a treatment for most pain problems. Usually we keep going until the pain settles. With chronic pain the pain remains, but the principle holds.

• Avoiding activities leads to weakness, stiffness, becoming unfit, boredom, amongst many other negative outcomes.

• If you pace successfully, you have a good chance of doing what you want without a severe worsening in your pain.

Trap No.5

"I let the pain guide me."

The pain will guide you right into a mess. When

you have little pain you are at risk of doing too much, when your pain is bad you may avoid. There is no future for you in this approach.

Antidote to Trap No.5

• Read this book carefully and put it into action.

Trap No.6

How you feel

We all tend to run our lives according to how we feel. Our moods have great influence over what we do and when we do it. That may or may not be ok in normal life but if you have a pain problem it is definitely not ok.

The whole point of pacing is to break the bonds of how your pain makes you feel and influences your decisions on activity. Using measuring, timings and quotas takes feelings out of the calculations. There's a reason for this and you know it by now.

Antidote to Trap No.6

• Again, stick to the principles. They may seem rigid and inflexible, but that's because we are so good at wriggling out of things we know we should be doing, in favour of things we would like to do! You can relax the rules later.

12

CHANGING BEHAVIOUR

Behaviour And Habits

OUR BEHAVIOUR IS what we do. Everything in human life is either a thought, a feeling or an activity.

Our behaviours are important and our most important ones are our habits. Most habits are good because they are useful. We have them so we don't have to think up a new behaviour every time we come across something familiar.

However, because they are useful and we use them so often they are set into our characters. This can make them difficult to shift if we want to.

This can give us two problems:

• We can have bad, or maladaptive, habits which we use again and again and which have the same poor results again and again.

• Habits are very difficult to change. Because they are habits!

My patients tell me that pacing is the most useful

thing I have ever taught them. Yet it's so simple, so what's the problem? Why can't everyone just catch on and apply the principles correctly?

Changing Our Behaviour

What are the hardest things in life to change? Your tax assessment? The colour of your carpet? Your car? Other people's opinions?

No! Your behaviour, that's what!

As we go through childhood and early adulthood we need to learn many behaviours to cope with what's going on in a complex world. These behaviours are useful, indeed essential, to our survival in human society.

We learn from those around us, our parents, other relatives, friends and teachers. We learn what we need to do in various situations to get a positive outcome. Once we learn these behaviours we repeat them again and again.

Most of our behaviours will suit the situations we encounter and we feel that things work out OK. If our normal behaviours don't work well then sometimes we try to change them to better suit the circumstances we are meeting.

Changing our behaviour is one of the hardest

things to do.

Does behaviour change matter? Sure it does. All the things that kill us these days are at least partly due to our behaviour.

We don't die so much these days from infections and diabetes. But from cancer, heart disease, strokes and road accidents. Smoking, overeating and driving too fast are just three things contributing to our medical ills.

But what's difficult about stopping smoking, dieting and controlling our traffic speed?

There are few more difficult things than changing an ingrained behaviour pattern and making a new one.

You know it's difficult to give things up and when you do it they don't always stay given up! So, you know it's important and it's going to be tricky. Later we will look at some ways of making your changes in behaviour stick.

13

TOOLS TO HELP YOU CHANGE

Change Is Hard

CHANGING IS HARD. And change is what needs to occur if you're going to make progress with your pain problems. It's useful to have some tools in your armoury to help you succeed.

The activities you're having trouble with are related to your goals. Your goals are what you want to achieve. To achieve them you often have to do things. Physical things such as sitting, driving, walking, bending, lifting and so on. So it's useful to get your goals straight before you start. Unrealistic goals mean you are more likely to fail in your task.

Making your goals into "good" goals often requires some work. The SMART checklist is a quick and easy series of questions you can ask about your goal to make it more effective.

Once you have your goal or goals sorted out, planning becomes important. Taking a bit of time to plan things out can make a huge difference to how things turn out.

Write Things Down!

It's easy to be vague about what goes on in our lives. What we want, what we intend, what we are going to do and not do. We can avoid being specific, or being precise, or facing up to failure by just not being clear.

One of the antidotes to this is to "write things down". I can't over-emphasise how important this is. Writing things down forces us to be specific, to put down in black and white what we intend to do and when. This is a good discipline as it forces us to be clear.

When we write things down, we commit ourselves to a course of action, and that makes it a little bit more likely that we'll go through with it.

When you write things down, make them specific, a bit like a recipe. If my recipe for Christmas cake was "put everything in a bowl, stir it round a bit and put it in the oven for a while", how do you think my cake would come out?

By being specific you create a recipe which someone else could follow and achieve the same results you are looking for. That means it's a clear plan.

If you are going to succeed, you are going to need to write it down at various stages. Showing your plan to someone else makes it more likely that you will go through with it. Consider sharing your plan with someone you know.

Goals

We seldom consciously think about getting things done. We just do them. And that is OK most of the time. However, if you are anything like me, you are not that efficient at doing all the things you should do or want to do.

Because you have a difficult hurdle to overcome, that of pain, it may help to define what it is you are trying to achieve. Otherwise, how will you know when you get there?

Goals give us a direction to focus our energy and increase our motivation to get there. Motivation is useful as pain is a powerful demotivator. You may have failed to increase your activity many times before so being motivated is crucial.

We have talked about increasing activity and you may have noticed we have not mentioned reducing pain as part of the plan. Any pain reduction will be welcome but it might be unlikely if you have had a chronic pain problem for some time.

If you put down pain relief as your main goal this may not be helpful. The chances this will occur are small, leading to failure, frustration and anger.

Focus your energy on achievable goals by going through the goal setting process. Write them down so they are clear to you and perhaps to others.

Long Term Goals

Long term goals are good but may not be the way to start your goal setting life. Long term goals tend to be larger and more complex and are better cut down into smaller goals.

Short Term Goals

Short term goals are best to start with. Several short term goals may add up to a long term goal. An example might be a longer term goal of going shopping. You can break this down into sitting in the car, being able to walk far enough and increasing your ability to carry light things.

It's better on average to set smaller and less interesting short term goals initially. This helps you learn the process and makes it more likely you will succeed. Success is important and builds on itself, so setting things up for success to start with is vital.

SMART system

Most of us are vague about planning new projects and the SMART system can keep us on the straight and narrow.

S For Specific

You have to be specific when you set your goal. "Getting fit" is not specific, neither is "losing weight", "walking further" or "doing more with the kids".

"I will go the the gym for 45 minutes exercise twice a week". "I will lose 12 pounds in 8 weeks" and "I will walk to the park and and throw a ball with the children on Saturdays". These are all much more specific goals.

One way of checking if your goal is specific is to ask yourself "If I gave this goal to someone else, could they do it?" If they could clearly understand what to do and when they should do it, then yes, it's specific.

M for Measurable

How will you know when you have achieved your goal? This is important for a feeling of self-achievement and is the reason for giving yourself a reward.

Some of the goals above are measurable. The gym attendance is 45 minutes, the weight loss will be 12 pounds, both these things are measurable.

Make sure your goals are measurable in some way.

A for Achievable

Your goal might be a good one for you but not be achievable for some reason. This could be pain, lack of fitness, the wrong time, problems with other people or lack of money. Make sure it is achievable or your goal may not be successful.

R for Realistic

There may be something you really want to do, perhaps something you did in the past and you think to yourself "Sure I can still do that."

But the reason you are reading this book is because things have changed and you are not as you were. Your goals and plans have got to be realistic for where you are now in your life, with your pain and the problems it brings.

T for Timed

Time may or may not be an important issue in your goals but it is useful to bring it into the mix as it makes some goals much tighter. If I have to lose two stone in six months I will know whether I have succeeded by weighing myself at that time point.

Putting a time element into the process adds a discipline which is useful. It gives yet one more way of nudging us towards a successful conclusion to our efforts.

When you have your goals and priorities clearly in mind and written down, subject them to the SMART test one by one. If they pass the test you are much more likely to get what you are aiming for – success.

Planning

So you've decided what it is you need to do and in what order you need to do things. Now we can move on to planning how you're going to do it. Planning is the HOW.

What's the point of planning? The only point is to make you more likely to succeed. This could mean whatever your goal is for the activity.

When we are doing small activities we do not usually need to plan, but even simple things like shopping can be more efficient if we make a list!

We would never dream of starting a big activity such as building a house or travelling across the world without a plan of some kind.

If you have pain then it's more difficult for you to achieve what you want so it becomes more important to plan for success. If you don’t then failure becomes more likely with all its painful and depressing effects.

Your plan should be specific and clear enough so someone else could do it without being uncertain. So “On Monday at 10 in the morning I’m going to walk for 15 minutes, sit down for 30 minutes then put my clothes in the washing machine.” would be a small plan but it’s very clear what has to be done.

Your plan should be like a recipe which has to be followed for the cake to come out best. And write it down!

Summing Things Up

WELL DONE!

YOU'VE made it through the book! I hope you have learned lots of interesting things about pain and coping with it. I have tried to give you a logical, clear approach to managing activities when you have a chronic pain problem.

I ask you to be open-minded when you read the suggestions I have put forward. You may think it all sounds a bit dubious and you couldn't possibly do things this way. This would not be unusual, many people think this at first, but find that in practice it works.

You always have a choice. I ask you to choose to suspend whatever feelings you have about pacing and try an experiment.

Take your worst pain-pushing activity and apply the Pacing System to it. Really have an honest go at it and see the results. Or, more accurately, feel the results.

It's hard but you can do it!

Thank you for reading my book. If you enjoyed it

or found it useful, would you please take a moment to leave me a review at your favourite ebook site?

Thanks!

Jonathan Blood Smyth

Connect with Me

I'd be happy to hear from you anytime, pick your contact method!

Follow me on Twitter at twitter.com/jonblood

Friend me on Facebook at facebook.com/jonathanbloodsmyth

Follow my blog at JonathanBloodSmyth.com

Favourite me at Smashwords at smashwords.com/profile/view/jonblood

FAQs

DO I HAVE to pace forever?

You may have to if you have a serious pain or disability. Your tissues may never be able to put up with strenuous physical work or long periods in one position.

This is part of the "accepting you are not as you were" idea.

Over time pacing can turn into a good habit and feel like much less hard work.

But the promise of pacing is that it is possible, with time and control, to increase your quotas. That way you can gradually, gradually do more of what you want.

How do I increase my quotas?

To start with, do not consider increasing your quota until you feel well in control with the level you are already using. That means you can do the activity successfully and regularly without badly worsening your pain. Once you have reached that level you can decide what to do next.

Do you have a go at increasing the time during the activity? Have a go and see how much you can do?

No, you are correct, this would be unwise! You have read enough to realise this is not the way I recommend.

If you get going with the activity and try and work out how much further you can manage while you are doing it you are very likely to overdo it.

When you have discovered how much is too much, it will be too late.

Take a sensible amount of increase which does not represent a large proportion of the quota amount and add it to your quota. Done! That's your new quota and you do not need my reminder to stick to it.

10% is a sensible level to increase to start with, though you may prefer larger or smaller increases for your particular tasks.

The good news is you may be able to continue increasing your quotas over time until they reach what for you might be reasonable times. Then you will be doing the maximum you sensibly can for the problems you have.

Has the 10% rule got any scientific backing?

No there isn't any good scientific evidence that a 10% increase in activity in THE right thing to do in pacing or in sport. We don't know what the right amount is and as everyone is different in so many ways I doubt there is one answer here. However, 10% is a good starting point and you'll get feedback quickly as to whether you've made the right decision. Then you can adjust up or down as you need. The amount for you will also vary over time so this reinforces the need to test and experiment gently to maximise your chances of getting it right.

Do I have to use a timer forever?

Not necessarily. Some people really like the timers or a stopwatch and use them all the time. Many have a vibrate mode you can use discreetly to time yourself in public and no-one will know.

Even better, you will learn to internalise the method. In other words your brain becomes aware of the correct amount of activity to perform automatically. Then you will stop at the correct times more or less and so will have total control over what you do.

Unless you are some sort of saint I do not expect you to observe these rules all the time. Some of you may even have families and jobs!

Few people can control exactly what they are doing all of the time. However, try and apply these principles as much of the time as you can. Many people tell us they have a better life because of pacing.

The ideal is: "During the last three months I have never stopped doing something because my pain was so bad. I always stopped because the time was up. And I'm enjoying life more".

Aiming for this is good although few of us may approach perfection in this technique. However, people constantly surprise me with how dedicated they can be to an idea once they find out how much it can benefit them.

What's the scientific evidence for pacing?

Pacing is not well represented in the medical literature and the evidence that exists is contradictory.

While there is some evidence of a connection between disability and avoidance of activity there is only limited evidence of a direct link between the two. Avoidance has been linked with poorer physical performance and poorer psychological function as well as higher pain levels. However all the studies so far have taken a snapshot of a group of people with pain and so we can't be sure which one thing is causing another.

Overdoing has been connected with increased disability in some studies and linked with increased ability in others. Keeping going with an activity in spite of the pain may be a positive way of coping, but excessive persistence can lead to severely increased pain and lower physical ability.

Some authors have suggested that the intent of the person towards pacing may be a key element. Pacing may be much better as an active strategy (to reduce disability and increase levels of activity) rather than a passive strategy (to avoid pain).

14

APPENDICES

Appendix 1. Action Plan

THIS IS A summary of the process of pacing, it seems long but is actually pretty quick once you get the hang of it.

1. Choose an activity you typically overdo and suffer pain afterwards.

2. Perform this activity until your pain STARTS to worsen. DO NOT go on as far as you can manage.

3. Record this length of time.

4. Repeat stages 2 and 3 a few times, at intervals.

5. Take an average of your readings.

6. Take 20% off your average.

7. Use this figure as the amount of time you do the activity.

8. Stick to this figure and DO NOT go over it. No excuses.

9. Leave at least twice your pacing time between

paced sessions.

10. Perform a suitable number of repetitions but do not necessarily try to complete the activity. When you do it well, reward yourself.

11. When you can do your pacing time easily, decide to increase your quota.

12. Increase the quota by a planned amount, not more than 10% of the total.

13. Use this increased amount as your new quota.

Continue the process until you feel you can do things as you wish or any more increases would worsen your pain.

Appendix 2. A Summary

THIS IS THE speed learning version of what you've just read.

1. Chronic pain is common and usually has no underlying medical seriousness.

2. Activities are often badly restricted.

3. Typical responses to pain are overdoing and avoiding.

4. Avoiding leads to depression and loss of fitness.

5. Fear of continuing damage underlies avoidance.

6. Overdoing leads to severe pain worsening.

7. Overstepping your tissue tolerances is counterproductive.

8. In time, overdoing can lead to increased disability.

9. Acute pain means it has come on recently.

10. Acute pain is often a warning of tissue damage.

11. Chronic pain is long lasting.

12. Chronic pain often does not indicate bodily

injury or damage.

13. Acute pain is useful, chronic pain is not.

14. Being guided by chronic pain is not helpful.

15. The central nervous system can amplify incoming pain messages.

16. If you overdo, the amplification can get worse.

17. Our behaviours are difficult to change.

18. You can choose a different way to behave if you want to.

19. Choose your worst pain-pushing habit, the one which hurts you most.

20. Measure how long you can do the activity before your pain becomes worse.

21. Take 20% off this amount.

22. Use this amount (80%) as a quota for the activity.

23. NEVER go over your quota at the time.

24. When you can do your quota easily and without pain consequences, increase.

25. Don't add more than 10% to your quota at any

one time.

26. Stick to your new quota.

27. Reward yourself for doing well!

28. Base your activity on what you have worked out and not on what you feel.

29. How you feel is a trap.

30. Beware of good days, you may be tempted to do too much.

31. Be aware of and counter the traps and obstacles before you start.

32. Use your self-discipline in this new way.

33. Go for it. In a planned way!

Appendix 3. An Example

YOU MIGHT FIND it useful for me to write out an example I have seen before.

Michael is house-proud and always tries to keep the family home shipshape. He does all the cleaning and managing of the household. He's the house husband and finds his neck and arm pain restricts his abilities.

On discussion with Michael, we have learned than ironing is one of the activities he has difficulty with. He has a family of five to look after so he can spend two hours doing the ironing several times a week.

When he spends too long ironing the pains are strongly increased, but he puts up with this and gets on with things. He feels it's weak to stop just because of pain, and besides, who else is going to do all the work?

Let's see what we can do to get Michael to pace ironing.

Teaching the pacing process

1. Michael measures the time he can iron for before the pain increases and he feels he would like to stop.

2. The average time this happens is after 20 minutes ironing.

3. 20 minutes minus 20 percent is 16 minutes.

4. 16 minutes is Michael's new ironing quota time.

5. Michael irons for no longer than 16 minutes at a time.

6. He leaves at least 32 minutes between sessions of ironing.

7. He does a sensible number of ironing sessions in a day. He has to work this out by trial and error himself.

8. When he achieves what he has set out to do, without overdoing, Michael rewards himself with a small glass of wine and a walk around the garden.

9. If he has worked out the times correctly, he repeats this process until 16 minutes of ironing gives him no pain reaction at all.

10. He decides to increase his quota by a minute and a half, to 17.5 minutes.

11. He continues with the process until he reaches a level he is happy with or finds he can not easily go beyond.

Appendix 4. My Pacing Worksheet

THIS SHEET IS designed to help you identify what you need to pace and find the appropriate activity levels for you.

The activities I tend to overdo and suffer after are:

1..................................

2..................................

3..................................

My worst pain-pushing activity is:

....

How long can I do this activity before I would quite like to stop, or my pain starts to become (significantly) worse?

1. Test time for this is ....minutes.

2. 20% of this time is ....minutes

3. Taking 2 from 1 equals ....minutes

4. Quota time is therefore ....minutes (same as last one!)

Do the activity to the number of minutes in 4 above, stopping when the time is up.

"Rest" in between sessions of activity for at least twice the time in 4 above.

Repeat until you can perform the activity in a controlled and repeatable way.

Consider increasing the quota (before you start the activity).

Make increase no more than 10% of the time in 4 above.

Add this increase to the time in 4 above and repeat the process.

Resources

HERE I'VE LISTED a few resources which cover the issues I have touched on in more detail.

Books

Manage Your Pain by Nicholas, Molloy, Tonkin and Beeston

This comprehensive book gives "Practical and Positive Ways of Adapting to Chronic Pain". Has ten 5-star reviews at the time of writing on Amazon (UK).

Overcoming Chronic Pain by Cole, Macdonald, Carus and Howden-Leach

"A self-help guide using Cognitive Behavioural Techniques" This book has 18 5-star reviews at the time of writing on Amazon (UK). Cognitive behavioural techniques are a powerful way of changing our thoughts and behaviour to allow us to move forward towards our goals.

The Challenge of Pain by Melzack and Wall

Although this is now dated it is a classic and worth reading. It does get technical in some parts and so can be difficult to follow but overall it is worth it. Has five 5-star reviews at the time of writing on

Amazon (UK).

Pain. The Science of Suffering by Patrick Wall

A review of pain from an expert researcher. Has five 5-star reviews at the time of writing on Amazon (UK)

Healing Back Pain, The Mind-Body Connection by John E Sarno MD, 2001, Grand Central Publishing

Dr Sarno has written a series of books on the connection between mind and body. He suggests that many musculoskeletal disorders are driven by subconscious aspects of our personality and that we need to address them if we are to have any hope of relief. With the increasing acceptance of psychological factors as relevant in many disorders, this is an interesting idea even if you don't take it literally to the extreme. This book has 106 5-star reviews on Amazon UK as of the time of writing.

Articles

(These are scientific articles, so technical++. You might be able to get them from a medical library, the British Library or its equivalent in your country.)

Activity Pacing in Chronic Pain, Nielson, Jensen, Karsdorp and Vlaeyen,Clinical Journal of Pain, Volume 29, Number 5, May 2013

Activity Pacing, Avoidance, Endurance, and Associations With Patient Functioning in Chronic Pain: A Systematic Review and Meta-Analysis, Andrews, Strong and Meredith, Archives of Physical Medicine and Rehabilitation, Volume 93, November 2012.

Website

The companion website for this ebook is Pacing For Pain.com.

<<<<>>>>

Printed in Poland
by Amazon Fulfillment
Poland Sp. z o.o., Wrocław

27403155R00081